HEART ATTACK AND BACK: TWENTY YEARS LATER

Heart Attack and Back: Twenty Years Later

Commitment to Wellness

Ross J. Giordano

iUniverse, Inc.

New York Lincoln Shanghai

Heart Attack and Back: Twenty Years Later
Commitment to Wellness

iUniverse books may be ordered through booksellers or by contacting:

iUniverse
2021 Pine Lake Road, Suite 100
Lincoln, NE 68512
www.iuniverse.com
1-800-Authors (1-800-288-4677)

Because of the dynamic nature of the Internet, any Web addresses or links contained in this book may have changed since publication and may no longer be valid.

ISBN: 978-0-595-45623-9 (pbk)
ISBN: 978-0-595-89924-1 (ebk)

Printed in the United States of America

CONTENTS

Preface

My name is Ross Giordano, and I suffered a near-fatal heart attack on May 2, 1987, at the age of forty-seven. If you've had a similar experience, I know your thoughts and emotions, because I have been there. My sole intention for this book is to offer hope and encouragement to anyone who has experienced the traumatic interruption of their life caused by a heart attack, heart bypass surgery, or heart disease.

Among the approximately 1.5 million heart attacks each year, of which approximately 600,000 result in death, you are among the survivors, and that is something you must be thankful for. Thankful may not be the most appropriate word considering your emotional and mental state, but you must consider that you do have the opportunity to achieve wellness in your recovery process. The degree of wellness you can achieve depends upon the severity of your disease, your physical condition, and your attitude.

Although everyone must contend with his or her own individual circumstances, your road to recovery should dominate your thoughts at this stage of your sickness. You cannot change what happened, but can look ahead to the fullest recovery possible by making the necessary changes in the life ahead of you. The road to wellness must start with a commitment to restoring your health, recovering, and planning for your recovery in consultation with your doctor. Be mindful of your own circumstance and your own healing pace. Accepting your present circumstance must be a prerequisite to your recovery journey.

You must now focus on attaining the highest level of wellness and preven-tion of future sickness.

Let the healing process begin in mind, body, and spirit with thank-fulness as you look ahead to tomorrow and the gift of life you will con-tinue to share with your loved ones.

Introduction

Although it has been quite some time since my heart attack, I still feel stunned when I recall that day and what happened to me and how it affected my family. I was in a state of anger. Why did this happen to me? Where do I go from here? What does the future hold? Can I recover? Can I go back to work? Can I still earn a living? Can I perform physically? How long can I live now?

Today, twenty years later, I am in very good physical condition largely because of my strong determination to achieve a condition of health far superior to my pre-heart-attack physical condition. I didn't know if that was possible when I was released from the hospital seventeen days after my heart attack. I reconciled my options and dispelled any fears of being handicapped. I made a mental investment that has resulted in my current physical well-being For myself and my loved ones, I chose a new lifestyle, a return to good health, and an appreciation of the gift of life and the caring of my physical well being for myself and my loved ones.

Twenty years later, I hold a strong conviction that heart disease is preventable through awareness of the causes, medical checkups, and a willingness and commitment to live a heart-healthy lifestyle. I believe that most—or maybe everyone of those who have experienced this sickness can return to a level of good health and an active lifestyle if they are committed to doing so and if their disease's progress allows it. Had I conducted my pre-heart-attack lifestyle in the same manner as my post-heart-attack lifestyle, I doubt I would have experienced heart disease.

If you have suffered a heart attack and want to prevent a second occurrence, there are certain rules you must adhere to regarding diet, and lifestyle. It is amazing to me how many of us think that heart disease only happens to other people. In fact, it only happens to approximately 1.5 million people each year, but that certainly could not include you, right? Let's say you are fifty years old and in ten years you will be sixty. In those ten years, there will be 15 million heart attack victims, 5.5 million dying from heart attack, but not you, right?

Heart attacks do not discriminate between male and female; approximately 50 percent of each will experience heart disease causing death. I was forty-seven years old when I had a heart attack; my neighbor was fifty when he died of a heart attack. In fact, three of my neighbors died of heart attacks in their early fifties. If you are among the millions of Americans who buy a lotto ticket—with odds of winning much less than your odds of having a heart attack—you'd better revisit your think tank. You think you can win the lottery, but you don't think you'll ever have a heart attack.

If you don't want to give up your current lifestyle, maybe you should give some thought to your family and loved ones who you would leave behind if you died suddenly, leaving your children without a mother or father, your grandchildren without a grandparent, your spouse without you or your income, or your parents, if they are still living, without a child. Heart attacks can happen anywhere and without warning. My neighbor who was in his early fifties collapsed from a heart attack while cutting his lawn and died before any help could arrive. Scary but true. Not to suggest that this disease runs in my neighborhood, but another neighbor of mine in his early fifties also suffered a heart attack, and upon his release from the hospital, he continued the lifestyle that caused his sickness. Three years later, he suffered a fatal heart attack while in a shoe store trying on a new pair of shoes.

Most heart attack victims experience warnings signs that should not be ignored no matter how slight. When a symptom arises, one must see his or her doctor immediately for a comprehensive and conclusive diagnosis. I am adamant on this, because we lost a family member who I believe would still be with us today had he received the medical attention he needed at the time.

By adhering to a heart-healthy diet, exercising, not smoking, controlling stress, controlling blood pressure and so forth, many heart attack victims have the opportunity for full health restoration. People in general do not have the desire to conduct a healthy lifestyle, perhaps because it is inconvenient, sacrificial, and requires leaving life in the fast food lane. They would prefer to indulge in the day-to-day pleasures of satisfying their taste buds and overdosing in laziness. If I have ruffled your feathers, you must be guilty of this.

Few people are concerned with good health until they lose it and become victims of heart disease, high blood pressure, and/or other related sicknesses. Even after a short recovery from an illness and a return to good health, they gradually gravitate to their old life-destroying habits.

Choose the path of a healthy lifestyle and you will be rewarded with a feeling of wellness, and, most likely, the absence of many types of sickness.

That Unforgettable Day

May 2, 1987, 8:30 p.m. I was at home. Mild chest pains bothered me, but I passed them off as indigestion. I went to the medicine cabinet for some Mylanta, which I was certain would relieve the pain. And why not? Only two years before I had experienced the same symptoms, and after obtaining medical attention, I was told I had indigestion and was prescribed Mylanta for relief. So this was just a re-occurrence, right?

Well, the pain did not subside. In fact, it became unbearable. I knew I had to act quickly and didn't want to alarm my wife. ("Uh, honey, I think I'm having a heart attack, but don't be alarmed." Right!) But I knew it was serious. I suggested she call the paramedics, which she did immediately. Sitting on the couch, I broke out in a sweat. Severe, crushing pains raged through my chest. I thought for sure the end was near. It damn near was, as a matter of fact. It seemed like an eternity before the paramedics finally arrived and attended to me, which I vaguely remember as I was in and out of consciousness.

Prior to being put on a stretcher and carried out to the ambulance, I was barely conscious and thought about what my wife was going through as she prepared for what was ahead of us. I remember her making many phone calls as the paramedics were attending to me, and although I almost passed out, I was mindful of the events around me and the scene I had created in the Giordano household. In and out of consciousness, I was put on a stretcher and loaded into the ambulance, then raced to the hospital with siren blaring, never thinking I would be a participant in this event, an event we have all witnessed so many times.

I was in the ER when I finally regained consciousness. I was administered an anti-blood-clot medication, which evidently relieved the blockage and allowed the blood to flow again.

Blood flowing is what it is all about.

A nurse asked me about the severity of the pain on a scale of one to ten. To the best of recollection, I believe I said seven. My heart had also lost its rhythm and gone into fibrillation and cardiac arrest. They used the paddles on me (I was told this later), which shocked my heart back into synchronization. During the time of my unconsciousness, I have vivid memories of puffy cloud formations with faces looking down on me and beckoning me to come. Just as vividly, I remember saying, *No, no, I'm not ready yet,* and suddenly waking up. This is truly a most profound memory. I believe I may have been between life and death and was coherent enough to discern between the two and denied death by choosing life.

As I slowly awakened, I prayed for my life and thanked God. I was so grateful to have regained a state of consciousness and to be coherent enough to realize what I had just been through. It was a frightening experience.

I remember my sixteen-year-old daughter, Lisa, whom they evidently allowed in the room, calling out, "Daddy, Daddy." I heard her, but I couldn't acknowledge her, as I was barely conscious. Upon awakening, while I was still groggy, a doctor stood at the foot of my bed and told me I had had a rough go and they had almost lost me. He said I might need a heart transplant, as there was severe damage. You can imagine the thoughts running through my head after hearing that. Shame on that doctor. Talk about bad bedside manner! That was entirely too much information at that time and place, and somewhat premature as well, for it turned out to be inaccurate. After hearing that, however, I was depressed and scared.

My mind was racing. First, I had a close call with death; now I believed I would be in the hospital for a long time, waiting for a heart transplant, away from work, an invalid, a handicap to my family, and so on. Although I didn't die, I thought life as I knew it was over. What a stressful time this must have been for my wife, especially after hearing this doctor say I would need a heart transplant due to the severe damage inflicted on my heart, definitely a premature judgment, as we later discovered.

Thank God for my father-in-law, who remained strong as he stood by my wife's side. My parents, who were in their late seventies, flew out from California. I felt angry for having put them through this at their age. I knew they were hurting inside, but they remained uplifting and encouraging at all times.

Loyola Hospital

I was admitted originally to a hospital close by, then transported to another hospital with better cardiac care. However, my father-in-law had me transferred again to Loyola University in Chicago, where doctors had the best expertise and equipment for treating me. Loyola is also a teaching hospital for heart disease and care. My father-in-law's supportive presence and assertive decision-making resulted in the best care and treatment for me, and I appreciate it still.

At Loyola, I underwent double bypass surgery. Normally this procedure uses a vein from the leg. They prepared my leg for the removal of the vein; however, my doctor chose to use a mammary artery from my chest. I had two blockages, one at 90 percent and another at 50 percent. It was the 90 percent artery blockage, a main artery, that caused my heart attack. An interruption in blood flow had caused so much pain, and it could have been fatal. The cardiologist later informed me there was some slight heart damage, but because the heart is a muscle, it could be exercised and made strong.

He said I didn't need a heart transplant, and despite the trauma to my heart, there was minimal damage. This was, without a doubt, the good news I needed to hear, and it inspired me to do just that: exercise my heart and make it strong. In my mind I had my life back now, and

I was focused on the future. I had a heart pump inserted to assist my heartbeat prior to surgery. Seventeen days in the hospital seemed like an eternity, a departure from the real world. I felt so out of step with life during my hospital stay. I knew hospitals were for sick people and I wanted out. I don't deny I was sick, but I embraced the thought that I could recover and make my heart strong again. What a positive mind-set this was for me and my family. You cannot imagine how good I felt knowing recovery was so near and so achievable.

During my recuperation, I recall gazing out my hospital room's window watching a nurse sitting on a bench eating her lunch. How lucky this person was to have life and health. I didn't know who she was or if she was really healthy, but the vision alone of this person was the perception of life and health.

Just a short time prior to my heart attack, I was engrossed in my job and all the triviality and stress it carried. Now, my work pales in comparison to the importance of the gift of life, health, and family.

Perhaps the girl sitting on the bench, eating her lunch, didn't harbor such thoughts of sickness, as people in general take life for granted. I suppose you need a serious setback to gain a sense of perspective and realize how precious life is.

In that one moment while I watched that girl, I committed one of the deadly sins: *envy*. I was envious of that person sitting on that bench enjoying the simplicity of life at that time.

How many times in our life have we faced some wonderful moments only to preclude the joy by not living in that moment with our mind elsewhere? Although I was uncertain how my life would unfold, I was comforted with the good news of my heart condition and determined to recover as fully as I was physically and mentally able as quickly as possible. Back to the simplicities of life which I now had a new perspective.

Only three days after my double bypass surgery, I lay in bed feeling pretty good. I wanted to wash my hair, sit on a toilet, and take a shower. After all, I was in the recovery mode, so why not? I disconnected my monitor and headed for the bathroom and a relaxing shower. Within seconds, my nurse apprehended me, scolded me, and led me back to my bed. This was a case of the mind leading the body, and it was not the first time.

I was very emotional during family visits, feeling I'd let everyone down and angry with myself for allowing this to happen. Anger was my strongest emotion during this time and even afterward. I was angry that others had to suffer emotionally. I was angry for the inconvenience I had caused everyone. I was never in denial; I felt empathy for everyone. I was angry that my job and all the stress it gave me was a factor in my heart attack. I was angry that I'd let my desire to my job with dignity, integrity, and honesty transcend my health. It was extremely difficult for me to accept what had happened, since I was only forty-seven years old, and I thought I was living a nightmare and would soon wake up. This sickness was only supposed to happen to older, or other, people.

My wife hid her emotions well, remaining strong, cheerful, and positive throughout this entire ordeal. So many episodes must have worked upon her emotions and nerves. For example, the morning I was taken to surgery, my wife went to the chapel to pray with my father-in-law. She was paged to come to the emergency room. I imagine her heart skipped a beat, and it must have been a long walk to that room, not knowing the reason for the page but imagining the worst. She was quite relieved when she arrived only to pick up my wedding ring, which they had removed prior to my surgery as a matter of practice.

Another time she was called to give her consent to a test that might prove fatal. My God, what trials she underwent. Comparatively speaking, I was the lucky one, for I was being administered to and cared for every moment, while my wife was left to her inner strength, resources, and of course her caring family members. They were not spared any grief throughout this ordeal. As much as my wife despised driving on the expressway, she bravely did this every day I was in the hospital. I believe we all have inner strength that lies dormant until called upon. The Holy Spirit is always with us and ready to help in every situation when we call upon it and trust it to see us through. We must acknowledge this presence, as we have this magnificent power and comfort at our disposal.

The day of my release was bittersweet—I was so thankful and grateful, so angry and remorseful. Guilt wrestled with joy. I left the hospital with a feeling of being reborn, but still I wondered: Would I ever be the same? The answer came quickly as I accepted my circumstances and promised myself to be better, stronger, and healthier. This was my commitment to me, my family, and my loved ones. I decided to focus on new expectations in my life. It was a new season for me and the promise of a sunrise, not a sunset.

ARRIVING HOME

Upon departing from the hospital, I realized I was about to begin a new chapter in my life, *A New Season of Sunrise*, and I was determined not to screw it up by letting trivial things invade my mental and physical well-being. Sure the job is important, but not when it takes a toll on your life. Contemptuous, you bet you are when you work hard, do things right, and get stressed out, only to find yourself out of work on Friday afternoon. Not long after my sickness, something happened called "company restructuring and re-engineering." It has happened to me more than once since my heart attack and I promised myself never to look back; companies that do this are not worth it. If you happen to encounter this, dismiss it immediately and get on with the importance of life.

Upon arriving home, my father reported that the garage door opener was not functioning properly. Well, here we go again—the mind was willing without considering the physical readiness of the body. I reached for the ladder, placed it under the garage door opener, and had one foot on the first rung when my wife scolded me down from the ladder. If you haven't noticed by now, I was the typical type-A personality. Mentally, all I wanted to do was resume a normal life as though nothing had ever happened. I was not handicapped and I was determined to get back in step with life even after this sudden and almost fatal interruption. Without realizing my circumstances, I was willing to jeopardize my new lease on life.

Well! I accepted my status unconditionally, meaning I would recover at the prescribed pace and I would fully resume all my previous activities (not lifestyle) and become even stronger without any limiting handicaps or restrictions. This was my course of action, mindset, and goal.

My cardiologist suggested I participate in a cardiac rehab program available at most hospitals. As good as I was beginning to feel, I realized this type of program could accelerate my plans to reach a new level of good health—I hoped as good as it had been when I was in the Marine Corps. I had a strong desire to restore my health and was determined to deny the impenetrability of short- or long-term illness brought on by my heart attack.

Cardiac Rehab

I joined a cardiac rehab program at a local college managed by a group of health professionals. The program included a very competent and knowledgeable staff and a variety of equipment. I was anxious to get started. The goal was to "return the cardiac patient safely and effectively to a productive and enjoyable lifestyle combining exercise, therapy and nutritional components." The program was directed by a board of certified cardiologists and administered by certified physiologist, dieticians, and registered nurses. They administered tests for blood analysis, body fat, muscle tone, lung function, and blood pressure. Each session ran one hour and was covered by my health insurance program.

I strongly urge anyone who is qualified for this cardiac rehab program to enter it with determination and commitment. If you work hard at it, you will experience well-being never felt before. Please discuss this with your cardiologist first.

When I arrived on my first day at the cardiac rehab class, I noticed people in various stages of health and recovery. My first thoughts were "What the hell am I doing here? This place is for sick people." I looked for someone around my age and saw men and women of varying ages. I needed to know if this happened to other people my age, and I quickly found out that heart disease does not discriminate by age or gender.

I needed to become an example to everyone, including myself, of how one can regain his health through a positive and willing attitude. I worked hard at restoring my health within the guidelines prescribed by the coaching staff. I needed to challenge my heart, strengthen it, and make it whole, since I had suffered slight heart damage. Since the heart is a muscle, I would make it stronger and repair the damage. I was motivated as hell to return to good health and maintain that good health.

I worked hard, and soon I was jogging three miles and feeling wonderful. I had a strong sense of achievement and pride. I never looked back. Please let me remind everyone reading this: when it comes to physical attributes, *I am me* and *you are you*. This was my achievement; yours may be different. Nevertheless, whatever you accomplish will be an achievement for you.

Diet and Exercise

Although I was mentally, and emotionally ready to return to work, I had to accept that physically, I had many weeks of recovery ahead of me. My body had undergone quite a shock and consequently required a period of rest and rehabilitation.

This was a most difficult adjustment for me, since I'm a type-A personality and never learned how to relax, but now I had to. Relaxation to me was doing something, not resting. A coworker of mine sent me a card that read, "Do not be anxious; let your body heal at its own pace."

During my rehabilitation, I did a lot of reading, especially books on health and nutrition. I had a real appetite for knowledge about what makes the body tick and, more importantly, keep on ticking. I especially wanted to know about the heart.

I discovered there were many trains of thought on the subject of heart health, and many things are still not known. Even now, twenty years later, we are still preaching diet and exercise for a healthy heart, which I enthusiastically believe and, of course, practice. Exercise is a key component to health restoration and longevity. Diet is also critical. A common-sense approach and a knowledge of the causes of heart disease will tell you which foods to eat and which foods to abstain from—

mostly which foods to abstain from. This, I believe, is the key to heart health with regard to diet.

Today, there are also many statin drugs for cholesterol control. These, however, carry many side-effects. Nevertheless, under certain conditions, cholesterol-lowering drugs may be necessary. You should work closely with your doctor to determine which one is right for you. I personally advocate diet and exercise for cholesterol control, unless you have a hereditary condition and require other means for maintaining low cholesterol. Even so, if you abandon diet and exercise and rely solely on drugs, your body is missing all the other benefits. These other benefits may prevent other illnesses.

Daily vigorous exercise, such as jogging, walking, or bicycling, can improve your health. You must raise your heart rate three to five times a week for twenty to thirty minutes to obtain the benefits. You're HDL (high-density lipoproteins), the good ones that remove cholesterol from your body, increase with exercise. Today, twenty years later, with all the knowledge we have gained, I advocate a well-balanced diet, daily exercise, low sodium intake, and weight control as the prescription for heart disease prevention.

You may wish to consider the Mediterranean diet. I believe it meets the criteria of a heart-healthy diet by providing the nutritional food balance our body requires. If you read the hundreds of books on heart health, you can't help but conclude they all basically deliver the same message: a heart healthy diet and exercise, which is also advised to prevent other illnesses such as stroke, cancer, and diabetes.

A heart-healthy diet is by no means doom and gloom for your food enjoyment. You can still enjoy *many* of the same foods as before, but you'll need to modify your diet to meet your body's nutritional and heart-healthy needs. You must reduce the frequency and portion size of foods that can cause sickness and heart disease, such as animal fats and other foods high in cholesterol, sodium, and sugars, which become triglycerides and part of total cholesterol.

Our family has discovered alternatives to ground beef, such as ground turkey for hamburgers, meat loaf, and tacos. Ground chicken would work as well. The addition of herbs and spices contributes to a tasty meal. In some cases, you may not be able to discern the difference between ground beef and ground turkey. Your taste buds can be fooled, but not your heart health. With my new regimen, a whole new nutritional world opened up to my family, which we continue to practice today.

Until you begin the exploration of a heart-healthy diet, do not be discouraged. Your life has just begun and you will benefit from these changes for a long time. Do not think about the foods you may have to give up; focus on what you can and should eat. You may be surprised at the options available to you.

The benefit of dark chocolate to heart health was great news for chocolate lovers. Nevertheless, remember portion size. Now is the time to invest wisely in the rest of your life. Your new diet is also beneficial for the prevention of a variety of other diseases, which you will learn about from the American Heart Association.

I am not a doctor or a nutritionist, nor will I pretend to be, but my answer to heart health, and for that matter good health in general, is simply a heart-healthy diet and sufficient exercise. If it is good for the heart, it must be good for overall good health as well. Avoid animal fats and any high sodium food or drink. High sodium contributes to high blood pressure and possibly other diseases. When you practice a heart-healthy lifestyle, your entire body benefits and you reduce the risk of other diseases.

Six Weeks Later

Within six weeks, I had returned to work, had resumed traveling on business, and, within sixteen weeks, was playing golf. I had felt physically and mentally ready to play sooner, but I had to wait for my stitched up chest to heal completely before any physical movements involving torque. What a great feeling to work and play golf. I had overcome this setback and was determined to become stronger and without physical limitation. *A positive attitude, strong desire, improved diet, and exercise. I was back—and loving it.*

I must add a word of caution: do not force the body to heal; it will do so at its own pace. I did challenge my body on occasion (part of my Marine Corp training), but I *mostly* stayed within the rehab guidelines, although I accelerated the schedule. In the early stages, I cried while jogging, so overjoyed was I by my progress. I challenged my heart when jogging, telling it, "Okay, let's see how strong you are." I ran hard, and I just kept running, recalling thoughts of my Marine Corp training, when we ran and hiked with full gear, rifle, and seventy-pound backpacks. We tired, but kept on, and when someone stumbled or dropped, we picked him up and helped him finish. We never left anyone behind and we never stopped until we reached our destination. But I am not advocating this to anyone. Please adhere to a disciplined rehab schedule and heal at your own pace. Anyone who has undergone any type of heart surgery and requires rehab must remember that we are all different when it comes to our physical and mental recovery recovery process. We have a body and a mind and for this assignment, they must be synchronized.

Do not dwell on being sick, but rather focus on returning to good health and always think positively, as this plays such an important role in the rehab process. Do not resign yourself to a handicapped lifestyle. Look ahead and see yourself in the condition you can realistically achieve. This is your goal—go for it. Do not surrender to being anything less than you can be.

Commitment to Wellness

Focus on Recovering to the Fullest

This must be your unwavering mindset and should dominate your thoughts. Join a cardiac rehab program right away. I urge you to do this, as you will derive numerous health benefits from the exercise programs, which will be suited to your needs. You will also enjoy the company of others who have experienced a similar sickness. Upon completion of the program, explore the possibility of continuance on your own, if possible. Do not terminate your exercise; it must be ongoing.

Commit to a Positive Mental Attitude toward Good Health

This is your daily mental mindset and goal; accept nothing less. You cannot change where you have been, but can change where you are going. If you are uncertain of where you are going, set realistic goals and commit to them. You are the captain of your ship and must chart your course to avoid sailing out on to choppy seas and putting yourself in jeopardy.

Begin and Continue an Exercise Program

This is an absolute must; be happy and thankful you can. Know your limitations. Even after your cardiac rehab program ends, continue an exercise program on your own in conjunction with your new healthy diet. Exercise is free and it benefits your overall health. You will feel good, look good, and live longer.

Watch Your Weight

Obesity is a major health risk factor. If you exercise and maintain a healthy diet, you can control obesity. Do not fall victim to a sedentary lifestyle. It is too easy; that's why most people embrace it. Do not become one of them. Give your easy chair and couch a rest; they will last longer, and so will you.

Maintain a Heart-Healthy Diet

Explore the many possibilities of nutritious foods and recipes. Eat heart smart. Do not think about what you may have to give up but rather the many new food choices you can discover. Please visit the American Heart Association Web site to learn about nutritional recipes, eating, and so forth. Also, visit your local bookstore, where you will find many books on this subject. Believe me, once you begin to eat heart smart, it will become part of your daily eating routine and you will be doing your body great benefit. This type of lifestyle will also put you in *sickness prevention mode*, protecting not only your heart but other parts of your body as well.

Do Not Smoke

Say goodbye to this dastardly, shameful, reprehensible disease-causing habit. Smoking is a desire of the flesh; do not let your flesh control your new, healthy lifestyle.

Control Your Blood Pressure

Normal blood pressure is an important component to good health. Read labels and watch sodium intake. I admit, I still use salt. However, I use it exclusively on popcorn and corn on the cob. That is the extent of my salt intake. There are many substitutes for salt that are not harmful to your health—explore them at your nearest health store. This is another health topic you will find on the American Heart Association's Web site. They provide information on high blood pressure, including its causes and how to avoid this life-threatening disease.

Have Regular Checkups

See your doctor. Do not wait until it's too late. Early detection means early prevention.

Live and Love Life (Perhaps a Second Chance for Some)

Do not be selfish. Share your new life with loved ones and become part of theirs. We must take off the blinders and become sensitive to and aware of our surroundings as life unfolds in front of us. Do not fear bad news from your doctor. Actually, any bad news can become fortuitous good news. Early detection, early prevention, and early treatment can save your life. Fear not the known but rather the unknown.

Try to Avoid Stress

Of all the above, I believe stress is the most difficult to manage. We face it daily and in many circumstances in our lives. In the same way that we have a choice of what foods to feed our body, we also have a choice of what thoughts to feed our mind. As tough as it is, we must nourish our minds with positive thoughts and dismiss anything we cannot control. We must walk away from stressful situations and let God take over and fight the battle. Hand it over to him and you will feel the burden lifted from your mind. Do not get caught up in the thick of thin things. (I have always liked this saying.)

I remember when I traveled heavily and worried about missing a flight or a schedule or a meeting. Thinking back about it, I know I put myself under stress for no good reason. After my heart attack, I adopted this thought: What was the worst thing that could happen if I missed a flight or a deadline? Putting these events into perspective helped me avoid a lot of stress in my life. Since my heart attack and (what I believe to have been a) near-death experience, I have met many people in the same circumstances and been astonished when I discovered they had resumed smoking, continued unhealthy diets, and refused to exercise. Earlier, I mentioned my neighbor. His attitude was that life was too short to give all this up, and besides, he had new plumbing, so he was good to go. This type of attitude epitomizes laziness, selfishness, and a lack of appreciation for life. It also embodies satisfying the desires of the flesh, which translates to mental weakness. When I questioned him about his attitude, he became very defensive and as much as told me to mind my own business. Perhaps I was naïve to think everyone held life as precious as I did. Well, it is twenty years later and he is no longer around. I am.

The greatest gift we have is the gift of life. To me, the meaning of life is simple: it is life itself, living life and enjoying all it has to offer. Think for a moment about your five senses and the enjoyment each one brings. Sure, we take this for granted and fail to capture the true essence of each sense. Sometimes we allow our senses to control our lives by yielding to them. For example, when we walk by the bakery and smell the cinnamon rolls, do we keep on walking or fold under the pressure of the aroma?

Accredited Visitors

Shortly after my heart attack and my return to good health, my wife and I joined the Mended Hearts organization. We became accredited visitors, meaning we were qualified for hospital visits to heart patients both pre- and post-op. This was a very rewarding experience, since we had a significant impact on patients we visited, who got to speak to someone who had undergone a similar illness. Seeing is believing, as they say. I recall the look on their faces during our visits; it echoed the thoughts I had during my hospital stay. Most importantly, they had someone who could understand, relate, and answer questions.

I believe we brought hope and dispelled many fears—fears of the unknown that I also faced. Foremost in my thoughts immediately after my heart attack were the questions, where do I go from here? What's in my future? How long will I live? Will I be handicapped? And so forth.

Shortly after my heart attack and subsequent return to work, I attended a meeting prefaced with small talk. The owner of the company was telling us about his tennis game. I mentioned that I would like to try playing tennis sometime, and he responded, "Can you do that?" Once again, I was motivated toward good health and was ready to challenge him to an endurance contest. It's funny how some perceive heart-attack sufferers as damaged goods. You may encounter this type of perception; do not let it fester and diminish your self-esteem. There are so many wonderful books and guidelines regarding this subject that there is no point in including this information. If you seek information on any of these subject matters, the American Heart Association has a plethora of free information—everything you will need to know regarding heart health, diet, exercise, and how your heart works. I urge you to contact them and obtain this helpful information. Also, you should seek out the local Mended Hearts chapter and join them for some friendly social support. Although it has been twenty years, I can still recall the entire process at Loyola, from arrival to going home.

Today, twenty years after my heart attack, I am in better physical condition than many people my age and many people quite younger than me, for that matter. I have seen many high school coaches who seem unfit to be teaching any kind of sport. You know what I mean. I'll bet they can't see the tips of their shoes when standing straight. What a poor example they must be for their students. I must admit, I still love my pasta and pizza and enjoy it frequently in conjunction with a heart-healthy diet. I just control the ingredients and portion sizes. "Everything in moderation" rings so true in all we do. By the way, the only medication I have taken since my heart attack is a coated aspirin, daily. It is your choice: reduce your life expectancy and leave your loved ones—or not.

Shortly after my recovery, many people were affected by what had happened to me and made their own lifestyle changes. You might say they got a wakeup call and a chance to evaluate their lifestyle. If you have found my story helpful, pass it along to someone you know who may be a candidate for heart disease. Do not be surprised if they refuse the advice or information. I wish you well. Feel free to contact me anytime. I would enjoy hearing from you. My e-mail: *rossi33@sbcglobal.net.*

My Motivation for Health Restoration, Sickness Prevention, and Longevity

My wife, Patricia, and children Lisa, Christina, and Joseph. Their spouses, Mark, Bryan, and Melissa. To be there for them and share our lives together. My grandchildren, Kyle, Jenna, Dominic, Mia, and Luca. Collectively, they are all my life and my greatest pleasures and treasures from God. Surely, you must have a desire to return to your best health for many reasons. Why not list a few?

- Resume life and all it has to offer

- Resume work

- Resume recreation

- Play with your grandchildren

- Teach your grandchildren about your special skills

- Be there for your children in time of need

- Take that special vacation with a loved one
- Explore your new lifestyle and all you can and should expect
- Read about the nutrition of foods and benefits of exercise
- Make new friends, join an association
- Perform volunteer work
- Start a new career
- Start a new hobby
- And much more

Heart Facts: Your Body's Engine

Your heart beats approximately 100,000 times in twenty-four hours.

Your heart will beat approximately 36.5 million times in one year.

Your heart will beat on average 2.5 billion times in a lifetime.

Your heart is approximately the same size as your fist.

Your heart weighs approximately seven to fifteen ounces.

Your heart pumps approximately 1 million barrels of blood in a lifetime.

The aorta artery is your largest artery and is approximately the diameter of a garden hose.

Your heart is located in the center of your chest and is slightly tilted to the left.

Your heart generates enough power in one day to drive a car twenty miles.

Your heart pumps about nine pints of blood per minute, 1,500 gallons per day.

Your heart is the hardest working muscle in your body.

Your blood circulates through your body 4,320 times in twenty-four hours.

Your heart's function is to pump blood throughout the body.

Your heart is a muscle designed for strength and reliability for one hundred years or longer.

The average man has between ten and twelve pints of blood in his body.

The average women have between eight and nine pints of blood in her body.

Stroke is the number-three cause of death in the United States, behind the number-one killer, heart attack.

Approximately 700,000 individuals annually are affected by a stroke.

Stroke is the leading cause of disability among adults.

A stroke occurs when an artery to the brain is clogged or bursts.

A heart attack occurs when an artery to the heart becomes clogged.

Your diet for heart disease prevention will also play an important role in the prevention of stroke.

It is just incredible to think about how important our engine of life, the heart, really is. It plays such an important role in society. Just think about the impact of one person having a heart attack and how many lives and entities, both professional and personal, are affected.

All heart health concerns the flowing of blood through the arteries without interruption. Perhaps not in my lifetime, but in my grandchildren's lifetime, a drug or food will be invented to keep the blood flowing. In the meantime, take care of your heart and keep that blood flowing.

GLOSSARY

Angina: chest pain due to an inadequate supply to the heart muscle.

Angioplasty: procedure with a balloon-tipped catheter to enlarge a narrowing in the coronary artery.

Aorta: the main artery and blood supplier of the body emerging from the left ventricle.

Artery: a muscular blood vessel that carries blood away from the heart.

Atrium: a chamber of the heart that receives blood directly from the vein.

Blood clot: produced by the body naturally to help stop bleeding when a blood vessel is broken or injured. Blood clots can sometimes form naturally and can be responsible for heart attack or stroke as they may clog an artery. If there is plaque buildup in an artery, there may not be room for the blood clot to pass, and they may block blood flow.

Capillary: a tiny vein (as thin as a hair) that delivers oxygen and nutrients to your cells.

Cardiac arrest: sudden and abrupt loss of heart function. The most common cause of this is coronary heart disease.

Cholesterol: A fatty substance (lipid) that originates from the liver and foods we eat.

Circulatory system: 60,000 miles of blood vessels (no kidding), including the heart (the pump), arteries, veins, capillaries, and lymphatic vessels.

Congestive heart failure: the inability of the heart to keep up with the demands on it, and the failure of the heart to pump blood with normal efficiency.

Coronary artery: an artery that supplies blood to the heart.

Coronary vein: a vein that receives blood from the heart muscle and empties directly into the right atrium.

Heart attack ("myocardial infarction"): this occurs when a section of the heart is deprived of oxygenated blood. A cause of this is when one or more of the coronary arteries supplying blood to the heart muscle is blocked. Blockage of an artery caused by the buildup of plaque (a fat-like substance) is described as atherosclerosis.

Heart disease: any disorder that affects the heart.

High blood pressure (hypertension): anything greater than 140 over 90.

Lipid: another term for fat.

Platelets: they help the blood to clot and stop the bleeding when a vein or artery is broken or a cut occurs.

Pulmonary artery: an artery carrying deoxygenated blood from the heart to the lungs.

Septum: the wall dividing the two ventricles of the heart.

Triglyceride: the major form of fat.

Vein: a blood vessel that carries blood to the heart.

Ventricular fibrillation: abnormal irregular heart rhythm.

Ventricle: a chamber of the heart responsible for pumping blood from the heart into the arteries.

SELF-ESTEEM

Self-esteem is all-important in your commitment to wellness and beyond. I was not going to discuss how you may be perceived in our society after a heart attack or any other heart disease. Unfortunately, this is reality, and you may at times be perceived as damaged goods. It is important that you turn a cheek and maintain your self-esteem despite the obstacles you will face. Some of the issues you may face if you are still a working person is how your co-workers and employers will look upon you. They may be sympathetic and consider you an unhealthy person, or a person who can no longer live a normal life, or a person who will have to drop out of the bowling league. In the eyes of many, you are no longer a whole person but damaged and unhealthy.

Even after two years of good health, many people asked how I was doing, which was okay. They showed empathy to a fault, as if to say, "Wow! You mean you can still do all those things?" I wanted to look them in the eye, tell them I was healthier than they were, and challenge them to a physical endurance test. It is a bitter pill to swallow, but it is reality and you must be prepared to deal with it.

Sometimes adults are just as guilty as children jeering other children suffering from a handicap. They can be ruthless and ignorant. This kind of behavior and perception is unlikely to change; just be prepared for how people look upon you and your sickness. This is the perception I faced prior to returning to work, during work, and afterward for many years. Frankly, it fueled my motivation to become healthier and whole again, to accomplish all that I did before and then some. I lost my job a short time after my heart attack, even after a return to good health with no handicaps or restrictions. The reason for my termination was company reorganization, so they say. I once overheard the CFO remark that I sure had cost the company a lot of money. My total hospital costs, including doctors, were over $60,000 in 1987. After my departure from the company, I had a difficult time finding a job within the industry. I felt certain it was because word got around about my heart attack and, as I said earlier, I was perceived as damaged goods, fragile and unhealthy.

It seems people derived some sort of pleasure broadcasting that "Ross had a heart attack." This irritated me, no doubt causing my blood pressure to rise. Nevertheless, I had to move on and control what I could, which meant moving on. I was more determined to get healthy, stay healthy, and ignore this shortsighted, small-minded type of thinking that permeates people's attitudes. I did find employment in an industry in which I was unknown. Eventually, I was hired back into the industry I left, never knowing if the president of the company that hired me was aware of my situation. We never discussed it, and he never brought it up, nor did I. I was healthy, performed my job without impairment, and just closed the door on that chapter, hoping it would not surface.

Although it was four years later when I returned to this industry, I ran into many people I knew while traveling to visit customers or attend trade shows; they often brought up the subject, but I quickly dismissed it, using the old cliché, "So, how is business?" They had the good sense to know I was not going there.

In closing, I wanted to give you this advice so you can be prepared for what may lie ahead of you. If you do encounter this attitude toward your condition, you do not have to endure it. Use it instead as a motivational tool and turn this hurt into a positive mental state. Rise above it.

Self-esteem is your weapon, which will melt away all the adversity and neg-ativity. Lock it into your head and throw the key away. You must claim ownership to your self-esteem and never, ever let anyone steal it from you.

The Gift of Life, the Meaning of Life

Ever wonder about this? I believe I found the answer when I almost lost it—life, that is. If you wish to know the answer, it's simple. Take a pen to paper and write down your answer to this question: What would I miss if I died tomorrow? Your answer will reveal the true meaning of the gift of life. Now that you know the answer to the question, I ask you, how much more meaningful is your health? I am sure your answers have given you new insights into your life, which you may have taken for granted.

I remember thinking of the times we went on vacation and I reminded myself of how enjoyable this vacation would be if I could bring my head with me as well as my body. You know what I mean. Although you may be spending time with your family or friends, your mind is elsewhere, usually on your job. I will never, ever again let my job steal these times from me, whether on vacation or elsewhere. Although I never made a physical list, I did make a mental list shortly after my heart attack, and at that time I realized how life itself was the center of my being, my universe. Life is like a book of chapters: if you lose a job, you go on to the next chapter. If you lose your life, the book has ended, for you have reached the last chapter. Knowing this helped me get through the tough times, such as the loss of jobs, for I knew that life itself was all-important and it gave me the hope and mental toughness I needed to deal with adversity. Today, I make it a point to live in the present so I may capture life as it unfolds around me.

Your List for Living

_____

_____

_____

_____

_____

_____

_____

_____

_____

_____

_____

_____

_____

_____

_____

_____

_____

_____

_____

Resources

Research regarding heart health, statistics, diet, and exercise has been taken from the following sources, found on their Web sites.

National Heart Lung and Blood Institute

NHLBI Health Information Center
Attention: Web Site
P.O. Box 30105
Bethesda, MD 20824–0105
Web: http://www.nhlbi.nih.gov/
e-mail: nhlbiinfo@nhlbi.nih.gov

Women's Heart Foundation
www.webmd.com
AMERICAN HEART ASSOCIATION
www.americanheartassoc.com
FDA Department of Health and Human Resources
Wwwmayoclinic.com
Healthinfo.org
Mayo Clinic Heart Healthy Eating Diet
Real Age Nutrition Center

978-0-595-45623-9
0-595-45623-5

www.ingramcontent.com/pod-product-compliance
Lightning Source LLC
Chambersburg PA
CBHW050340290526
45785CB00006B/2569